Dr Brian's

How To

Reduce Cholesterol

Naturally

All you need to know about fatty acids, healthy cholesterol levels and hardening of the arteries

ISBN-13:
978-1489580528

ISBN-10:
1489580522

ABOUT THE AUTHOR

My name is Dr Brian. I am a medical doctor with over 30 years experience and have been specialised in Nutritional Medicine for over 10 years. I am a *cause-orientated* doctor and much prefer the use of natural remedies wherever this is both possible and effective. I have helped countless numbers of people reduce their raised cholesterol and triglyceride levels naturally, without the use of statin or other drugs.

Many people already on statins have managed to either reduce or stop their use of these drugs safely. Much of the information in this book has been gained through my personal experience in successfully dealing with many difficult cases of hyperlipidaemia.

CONTENTS

Understanding fatty acids, triglycerides, cholesterol and lipoproteins

What are LIPIDS?

Both cholesterol and triglycerides fall into a category of naturally occurring fat molecules called Lipids. Also included in this list are waxes, sterols, fat-soluble vitamins (such as vitamins A, D, E, and K) and phospholipids.
They can be drawn as diagrams using the following letters;
C = Carbon
O = Oxygen
H = Hydrogen

Oils are simply liquid fats.

What are FATTY ACIDS?

These are chains of carbon atoms (-C-C-) of varying length with a COOH (the so-called carboxyl group, which is *fat soluble*) at the beginning of the chain ('alpha' end) and a CH_3 (the *so-called* methyl group, which is *water soluble*) on the other end, which is called the omega (meaning 'last') end.

Fatty acids can be;

1. **Saturated** (each carbon atom in the chain is saturated with hydrogen atoms and the carbons are all linked by single bonds). These fats are *solid* at room temperature. They look like rowing boats!

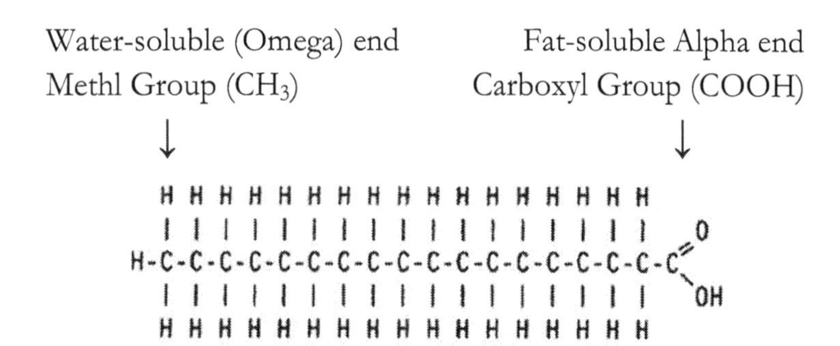

Examples of foods containing saturated fats are red meat, chicken skin and butter.

2. **Mono-unsaturated** (one double bond is created between two carbon atoms in the chain when hydrogen atoms are lost). These fats are *liquid* at room temperature. An example is olive oil. See the one double bond (-C=C-) in the middle?

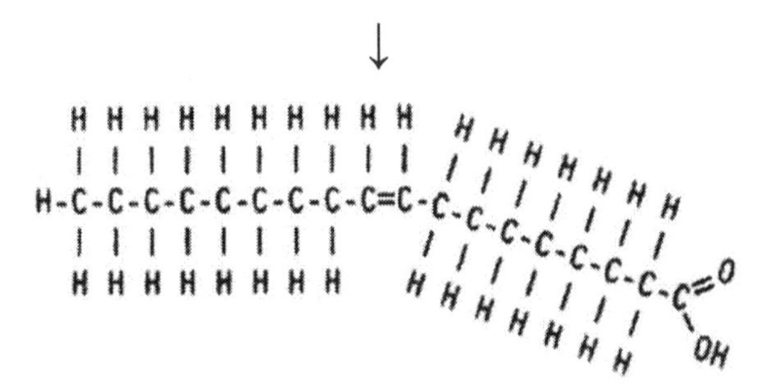

3. **Polyunsaturated** (more double bonds are created in the chain). These fats are also *liquid* at room temperature. Examples include fish oil, sunflower oil, flax seed oil and evening primrose oil. So you have seen that when hydrogen atoms get removed from the carbon atoms in the chain (they become less saturated with hydrogen = unsaturated), and double bonds are created. The more unsaturated the fatty acid becomes, the more double bonds there are.

The position of the *first double bond from the omega end* of the chain (the last carbon atom) dictates whether the fat is an omega-3 (three carbon atoms from the end, or omega minus three) or omega-6 (six carbon atoms from the end, or omega minus six). If you look at the diagram of olive oil you will see that the first double bond is at the ninth carbon from the omega end, making it an omega-9 oil.

Omega-3: **(count the carbon atoms from the left side = 3, then the first double bond appears!)**

↓

```
  H H H H H H H H H H  H H H H H H H H H
  | | | | | | | | | |  | | | | | | | | |     O
H-C-C-C=C-C-C=C-C-C=C-C-C=C-C-C=C-C-C-C-C//
  | | | | | | | | | | | | | | | | | | |    \
  H H H H H H H H H HH H H H H H H H H      OH
```

Examples of foods containing omega-3 oils are oily fish, linseeds (flax seed), rape seed (canola oil), soybeans and corn. The most important oily fish are salmon, mackerel, anchovies, sardines/pilchards, herring and tuna.

Omega-**6**: (6 carbon atoms from the left before the first double bond appears!)

↓

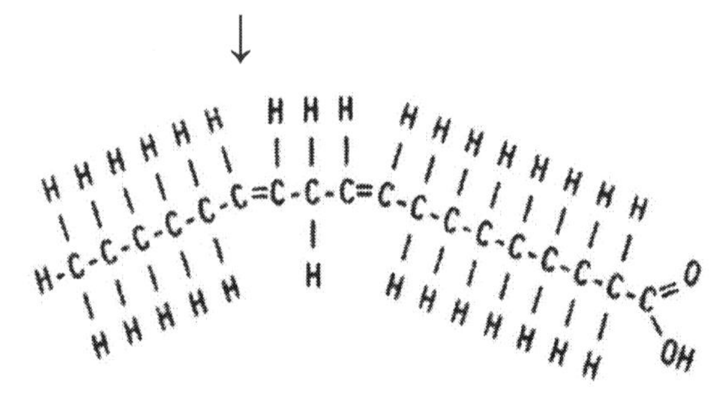

Examples of foods containing omega-6 oils are sunflower, safflower, sesame seeds, cotton seeds, oats, borage, blackcurrant and evening primrose oil.

4. **Hydrogenated** (processed) fats and **Trans** fats. If you have a *liquid* polyunsaturated fat and you want to solidify it (e.g. turning corn oil into margarine), you have to hydrogenate it, i.e. fully or partially saturate it with hydrogen. You normally achieve this by heating it up and adding pressurised hydrogen gas together with a nickel catalyst. The resulting margarine, which is *solid*, is then called a hydrogenated fat.

If the process of hydrogenation is partial, i.e. the resulting fatty acid is not fully saturated with hydrogen, one hydrogen atom can move to the opposite side.

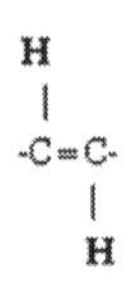

The resulting unsaturated fatty acid is called a **trans**-fat.

The level of saturation determines whether the fatty acids will increase or reduce cholesterol levels;

- Saturated and Hydrogenated fats *increase* cholesterol, and
- Unsaturated fats (Mono- or Poly-) *decrease* cholesterol.

There are two main types of fatty substances in our blood;

1. Triglycerides and
2. Cholesterol, which is further divided into various groups, the most important being;
   LDL or 'bad' cholesterol, and
   HDL or 'good' cholesterol,
   both of which we will discuss later.

Triglycerides

The structure of triglycerides (TG) is quite different from that of cholesterol. Each molecule is made from one molecule of glycerol and three fatty acids, looking like a capital E.

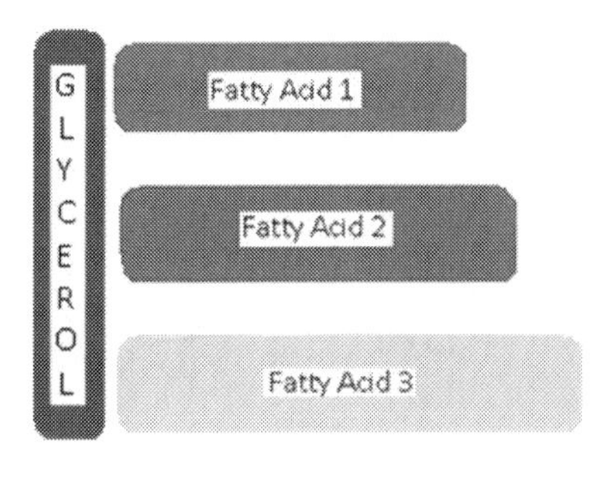

Each fatty acid in the molecule can be either saturated, mono-unsaturated or poly-unsaturated.

Hypertriglyceridaemia

Normal levels of triglycerides in the blood are lower than 1.7 mmol/l. Hypertriglyceridaemia is a condition where the blood levels after an overnight fast are above 1.7 mmol/l. This is important because high levels are a risk for developing cardiovascular (heart) disease.

Causes of Hypertriglyceridaemia;

- Consuming *excessive amounts* of alcohol, dairy products, meat, fatty foods and refined sugars (cane sugar, sweets, cakes, biscuits)

- Being *overweight*

- Being *over-produced* by the body's fat stores or liver.

- Having *diabetes mellitus* (types 1 and 2)

- Having a *genetic* predisposition or tendency to having high triglycerides, and

- The use of *medications* such as steroids, beta-blockers, thiazide diuretics, tamoxifen and oestrogen.

The treatment is going to be based on the cause. This sensible approach should be adopted more broadly in medicine, rather than relying totally on prescription medicines. The natural management of hyperlipidaemia is discussed later.

Cholesterol

Cholesterol is a type of fatty substance in the body that is *essential for healthy living.* Only levels raised above the norm and those that have been attacked by free radicals (see later) are harmful.

In 1967, François Poulletier de la Salle first identified cholesterol in solid form in gallstones. The name originates from the Greek '*chole*'- (bile) and '*stereos*' (solid), and the chemical suffix –'*ol*' indicating an alcohol group or OH at one end. It was only in 1815 that the chemist Eugène Chevreul named the compound "cholesterine", which we call cholesterol today.

The body absorbs, manufactures and uses cholesterol in order to carry out important bodily functions, which we will discuss shortly. Although cholesterol is absorbed from the diet, the majority of the cholesterol in your blood stream comes from being produced in the liver! It has been estimated that 10-30% of the cholesterol in the bloodstream comes from the diet, and 70-90% from being produced in the liver.

As you can see in the diagram, the cholesterol molecule is much larger than fatty acids and triglycerides. It has a similar carbon backbone or chain, but in addition there are a number of ring structures attached at one end. There is no such thing as saturated or unsaturated cholesterol as there is with fatty acids.

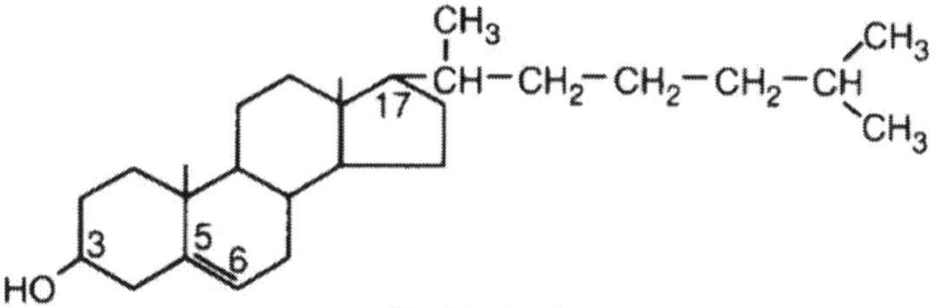

Cholesterol

The **benefits of cholesterol**;

- It is an essential component of our cell membranes, where it is required to establish proper membrane permeability and fluidity.

- Cells need cholesterol to help them adjust to changes in temperature. It is also used by nerve cells for insulation.

- Cholesterol is essential for synthesizing (making) a number of critical hormones, including the stress hormones (cortisol and dehydroepiandrosterone [DHEA]) and the sex hormones (testosterone, progesterone and oestrogen).

- Cholesterol is an important component in bile, a fluid produced by the liver that plays a vital role in the processing and digestion of fats.

- Your body also needs cholesterol to make vitamin D; in the presence of sunlight, cholesterol is converted into vitamin D.

- It aids in the absorption of fat-soluble vitamins A, D, E and K.

- The brain is the most cholesterol-rich organ in the body. A whopping 25% of all our cholesterol is found in the brain[50]. Cholesterol is important for the proper functioning of synapses – areas where nerve cells communicate with one other, and is important for the growth and repair of the myelin sheath (protective wrapping around nerve axons)[50]. Cholesterol also helps maintain serotonin levels.

- Cholesterol is a source of fuel, burnt to make energy.

- Cholesterol restores muscle mass and increases muscle strength during resistance training.

The known dangers of low cholesterol

We need to dispel the myth that 'cholesterol is bad'. Even though we have knowledge of the benefits of cholesterol, a common experience for us is to be told that we need to get our cholesterol levels as low as possible. Such advice can be dangerous to your health! We need to respect the reasons why we have and need cholesterol as well as the dangers of having levels too low. Various trials have shown that **low levels** of cholesterol have been associated with an increased risk of cancer[7], memory loss[13], dementia[14], depression[9] (due to low serotonin), suicide[15] and haemorrhagic strokes (bleeding, not blockage). In addition, two cholesterol agents (simvastatin and ezetimibe) taken in combination may increase the risk of cancer[39]. Modern research is showing the importance of normal cholesterol levels in preventing Alzheimer's Disease[50].

So, ***it's all about balance***! Not only do we need balanced levels of cholesterol, but also balanced attitudes to cholesterol in terms of its benefits and its dangers. Few experts would disagree that very high levels of cholesterol can be harmful, but please let's not drive levels into the ground either.

Now we will look at the dangers of having high cholesterol.

Hypercholesterolaemia

This is a condition where the blood level of the total cholesterol is increased above the normal of 5.0 mmol/l after an overnight fast.

Causes of high cholesterol:

1. High cholesterol tends to run in families. *Familial hypercholesterolaemia (FH)*, which is an inherited (genetic) problem of overproduction of cholesterol in the liver with grossly elevated LDL ('bad' cholesterol, see later) levels in the blood, resulting in premature atherosclerosis (hardening of the arteries, see later). Only 14% of the estimated 110,000 of cases in the UK have been diagnosed. It affects 1 in 500 people in the world. There is a 50% chance of passing it on to each child. The gene on chromosome 19

that codes for LDL receptors on cell membranes is faulty, resulting in either too few or inefficient LDL receptors, making them unable to remove LDL cholesterol from the blood. In the liver this causes a drop in LDL uptake from the blood (because there are too few receptors there as well), resulting in an even greater production of cholesterol by the liver. This is because the liver falsely detects low cholesterol and responds by boosting production[44].

2. Consuming excessive amounts of *saturated fats* (animal meats, chicken skin, sausages, bacon, liver patè, hamburgers, cheese, milk, butter, cream, ice-cream, chocolate, fudge, toffees, cakes, biscuits, pastries, creamy sauces, mayonnaise, coconut oil, palm oil, chips, crackers, cookies). Saturated fats ↑ total cholesterol and LDL.

3. Consuming too many *foods high in cholesterol.* Because cholesterol is produced by the liver, only animal products have cholesterol, e.g. meat, liver, liver patè, kidneys, poultry, shellfish (not fish), egg yolk and dairy products such as cheese, cream and butter.

4. *Hydrogenated* fats (e.g. most margarines) raise cholesterol just as much as saturated fats[30].

5. Consuming foods high in *refined carbohydrates* (sugar, cake, sweets, biscuits, white bread, crisps, ice-cream, sugar-sweetened drinks).

6. An underactive thyroid (*Hypothyroidism*). Here, the rate of metabolism is decreased and less cholesterol gets burnt for energy and heat production.

7. *Age and sex.* Prior to their menopause, women usually have lower total cholesterol levels than men of the same age. After about age 50 years, postmenopausal women often have higher total cholesterol levels than men of the same age. Cholesterol levels rise in both men and women until the age of 60-65 years.

8. *Stress* is only a cause in that it adversely affects eating and lifestyle habits.

9. *Alcohol* use: Moderate intake of alcohol (1-2 drinks daily) increases HDL ('good' cholesterol) but does not lower LDL ('bad' cholesterol). Excess drinking can also raise triglyceride levels, damage liver and heart tissues, and cause high blood pressure. This is why the habit of drinking alcoholic beverages should not be used as an excuse to prevent heart disease.

10. *Coffee* can increase cholesterol if it is not filtered [34].

11. *Low levels of vitamin C* have been linked to high cholesterol and low HDL (good) cholesterol. However, it appears that vitamin-C will only lower total cholesterol and increase HDL if levels are very low to start with [49].

If we are going to be cause-orientated in our management planning, we need to consider why levels of cholesterol are raised within each individual and not treat everybody in the same way. This targeted approach is far more satisfactory for both the patient and the doctor!

Lipoproteins

We all know that fat (and oil) doesn't dissolve in water. The bloodstream is mostly made up of water, so how are fatty acids, cholesterol and triglycerides transported around the body?

Nature (as usual) comes up trumps by attaching the fats to water-soluble proteins. The fat and protein together form spherical (ball shaped) objects called lipoproteins. The *proteins are situated on the outside* of the ball, while the *fats are carried inside*, away from contact with the blood. The lipoproteins are then able to transport the fats properly suspended in the bloodstream. In addition, the outside of the sphere has different apoproteins, which dictate whether fats are deposited in the walls of blood vessels, or carted away. This is more or less what they look like;

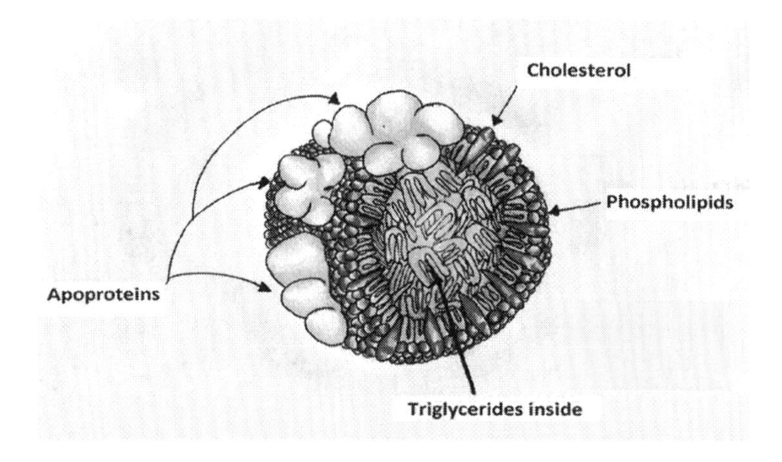

There are two main types of lipoprotein:

- LDL (low-density lipoprotein) – the potentially **harmful** type of cholesterol, also known as "bad cholesterol", and

- HDL (high-density lipoprotein) - a **protective** type of cholesterol, also known as "good cholesterol".

While LDL delivers its cargo of cholesterol to tissue cells, some is oxidised by free radicals (this is bad) and then deposited in the inner lining of the arteries, causing them to narrow and weaken (this is called atherosclerosis, see pg 20).

On the other hand, HDL cannot deliver cholesterol to tissue cells. Instead, it has the ability to scavenge deposited oxidised cholesterol from the lining of the arteries and return it to the liver for recycling or excretion in the bile.

Think of LDL as the cholesterol delivery truck and HDL as the pick-up truck! Another way of seeing it is that HDL is the broom, sweeping the dirty LDL away. Having too much LDL cholesterol in your blood can increase your risk of getting cardiovascular disease (e.g. atherosclerosis, angina & heart attacks), as well as strokes. The risk is particularly high if you also have a low level of HDL cholesterol.

We should not be too dogmatic about LDL as only being 'bad'. It has been shown to have some beneficial properties, such as being able to neutralise bacterial toxins, e.g. α-toxin produced by Staphylococcus aureus[47]. There will also be other benefits from LDL that we don't know about yet.

The functional difference between LDL and HDL results mainly from the different character of their surface *apoproteins*. LDL has apoB-100, which allows for the delivery of cholesterol to tissue cells by binding to receptors called LDLR. HDL has apoA-1, which allows for the scavenging of cholesterol. We need to have optimum levels of 'good' HDL in order to scavenge (remove) 'bad' LDL from arterial walls.

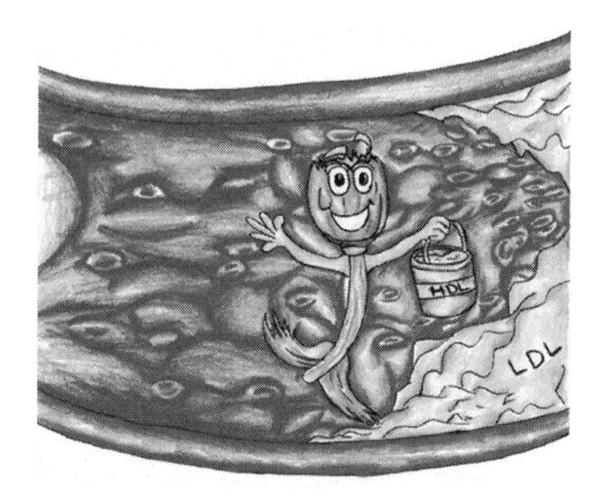

Another way to look at this is; "The **L**DL should be **L**OW and the **H**DL should be **H**IGH".

What should the various cholesterol levels be?

Remember the phrase "*Strive for 5*" when thinking of the total cholesterol level. However, doing a total cholesterol on its own doesn't tell us about the LDL and HDL values. It is perfectly possible to have a normal total cholesterol, but high LDL and low HDL levels. For this reason it is better to do a fasting lipogram (lipid profile), which includes total cholesterol, LDL, HDL and triglyceride levels, as well as the ratio of HDL to the total.

The 5-3-1 rule

Total Cholesterol (TC)[27] should not be more than **5** mmol/l.	**Levels > 6.2 = high risk.**
LDL[27] should not be more than **3** mmol/l	**Levels > 4.9 = high risk.**
HDL should be above **1**.	**Levels < 0.9 = high risk.**

Triglycerides should be less than 1.7mmol/l.

The ratio of total cholesterol to HDL (TC:HDL) should be less than 5 in men and less than 4.5 in women.

HDL can also be expressed as a percentage of the total;

HDL > 40% of total cholesterol = excellent

HDL > 30% of total cholesterol = ideal

HDL< 20% of total cholesterol = increased risk

If you have diabetes or a family history of heart disease you should consider targeting a somewhat lower level than the TC of 5 and LDL of 3 .[28] However, remember that very low levels are to be avoided (see 'Benefits of cholesterol' on page 8 and 'dangers of very low cholesterol' on page 9). In my opinion, total cholesterol levels should be between 4 and 5 mmol/l.

We will see later how to manipulate HDL upwards and LDL downwards, even if total cholesterol levels are within the normal range.

The flow of fats around the body

This section is for the more scientifically minded. The body utilises (can process) approximately 1000mg cholesterol a day.

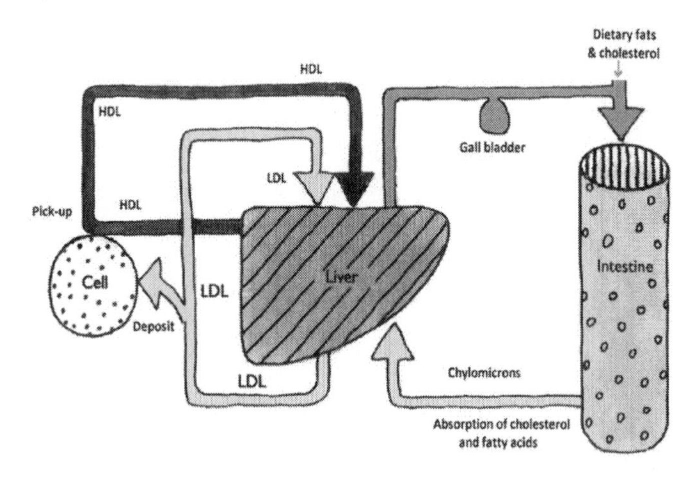

We saw earlier that only 10-30% of blood cholesterol comes from the diet. The other 70-90% is synthesised (manufactured) by the liver.

The fats we eat get absorbed in the intestines and then get transported to the liver as part of large, fat-rich lipoproteins called chylomicrons (see diagram). These lipoproteins are different to LDL and HDL. Once inside the liver the fats are changed into the two types of fatty substance, namely cholesterol and triglycerides.

From the liver, the cholesterol and triglycerides are pushed out into the bloodstream in the form of very low density lipoprotein (VLDL), which are worked on by the enzyme cholesterol ester transfer protein (CETP), which makes the lipoproteins more and more densely packed until they become low density lipoproteins (LDL). At the same time they lose fats to the tissues to be used and to fat stores for storage. In the process they become smaller and denser. The loss of fats from lipoproteins is through the action of the enzyme lipoprotein lipase, which is found on the surface of endothelial cells (inner lining) of the capillaries.

The liver makes bile, which is very rich in cholesterol. The bile flows into the gallbladder and from there into the intestines. Approximately 90% of the cholesterol in bile is then reabsorbed into the bloodstream within chylomicrons. This is an important concept to understand because *trapping* cholesterol in the intestines so as to prevent re-absorption will be a major strategy when we get to treatment.

How do statins work?

In the liver there is an enzyme with a very long name called 3-hydroxy-3-methylglutaryl coenzyme-A reductase (HMG Co-A reductase), which is required for cholesterol manufacture. It is more active at night. Statin drugs work by suppressing this enzyme and that is why they are normally taken at night.

However, HMG-CoA reductase also produces **Coenzyme-Q10** (CoQ10). We can then understand how taking statin drugs will cause a reduction in our levels of CoQ10.

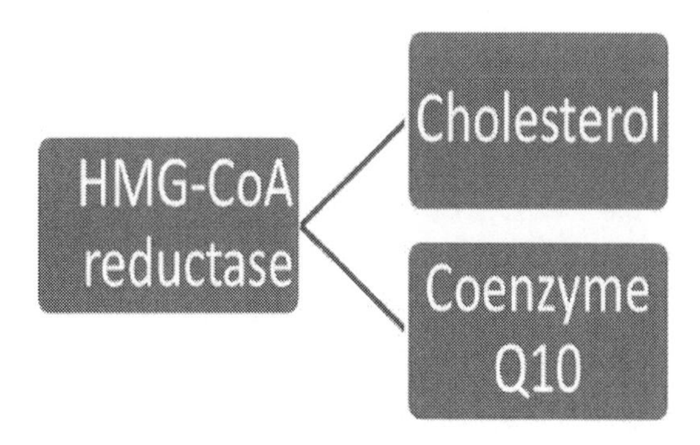

Why is CoQ10 so important?

1. It is vital for the production of energy by every cell in the body. The heart muscle requires four times more Co-Q10 than any other muscle or cell.

2. It improves muscle function (especially the heart muscle).

3. It is a fat-soluble antioxidant (neutralises free radicals). This means that Co-Q10 helps to prevent damage to our tissues by free radicals (the things that cause ageing, cancer, inflammatory diseases and many other undesirable conditions).

4. It rescues distressed cells in the major organs, bones, skin, hair, nails and eyes.

Our organs may become impaired (unable to work properly) if CoQ10 falls by 25 percent. Very low levels can even cause death.[21,22]

This is why I like to advise everyone taking a statin drug to consider taking Co-Q10. The exception occurs with those taking coumarin (Warfarin) because Co-Q10 is CONTRA-INDICATED (cannot be taken) with Warfarin! This is because it reduces the absorption and/or bioavailability of Warfarin, which can be dangerous! In such a case it is important to use the lowest dose of statin possible and to follow all the other advice found in the Natural Treatment section from page 24.

Co-Q10 should be used with caution in people taking certain other drugs, e.g. doxorubicin, gemfribrozil, perphenazine, propranolol, thioridazine, timolol and tricyclic antidepressants, e.g. Amitriptyline. The dose of Co-Q10 may need to be adjusted in these cases.

What is Atherosclerosis?

Some people call this "hardening of the arteries". This is a type of cardiovascular disease that begins with the deposition of oxidised LDL (damaged by free radicals) in the inner wall of blood vessels. This causes inflammation and the deposition of more cholesterol and the formation of scar tissue. This then hardens into a 'plaque'. Plaques increasingly narrow the blood vessel, reducing the flow of blood (and oxygen) to the organs. In the brain this causes strokes. In the heart it causes angina (chest pain, particularly during exercise), and coronary thrombosis (heart attack).

There are three processes involved in the formation of atherosclerotic plaque;

- Raised levels of LDL cholesterol,

- Injury to the arterial wall's endothelial (inner) lining, causing **inflammation**, and

- High levels of **free radical**s (as opposed to antioxidants), causing LDL to become oxidised (damaged) and taken out of the system by being placed in plaque.

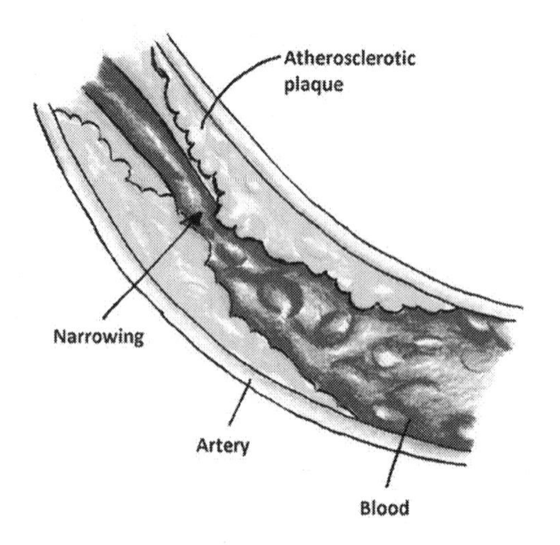

Cardiovascular disease is the main cause of death in the UK with almost 200,000 cases occurring per year. Studies have shown that 2 out of 3 adults in the UK have more cholesterol in their bodies than is recommended[29]. Lowering high cholesterol levels has proven beneficial in terms of reducing cardiovascular disease. Some opponents to the theory that "high cholesterol causes heart attacks" say that high cholesterol alone cannot be the cause of heart attacks because about 70% of people that have heart attacks have normal levels of cholesterol. We have already seen that there are three processes involved in the narrowing of arteries on page 21, but it would be helpful to know what the actual risk factors are for developing cardiovascular disease.

Risk factors for cardiovascular disease;

- Raised levels of LDL cholesterol, particularly when HDL cholesterol levels are low
- Diabetes mellitus (type 1 and 2)
- High blood pressure (hypertension)
- Being overweight and inactive
- Smoking
- Elevated levels of platelet-activating-factor (PAF)
- Elevated levels of homocysteine
- Elevated levels of C-reactive protein (CRP)

- Low levels of Coenzyme-Q10

The Natural Management of Hyperlipidaemia, Hypercholesterolaemia and Hypertriglyceridaemia

The sensible approach is always going to be to first **assess the causes** and **risk factors**. The chosen plan should be *tailor made* for the individual, their dietary and lifestyle habits, other medical problems (e.g. thyroid, liver and kidney disease, raised homocysteine levels, high blood pressure), their family history of heart disease, their lipogram readings and even their pocket (some products are expensive).

My approach is as follows;

Assess other risk factors

Assess other risk factors for cardiovascular disease, such as high blood pressure (hypertension), obesity, diabetes, family history of heart problems or stroke, early menopause, smoking, stress (leads to snacking on the wrong foods), raised fasting homocysteine levels, raised CRP levels (indicator of heart disease) and low levels of Coenzyme-Q10.

Thyroid Hormones

Have thyroid hormones checked; low thyroid function is one cause of raised blood cholesterol. This is because less cholesterol gets burnt to provide energy and heat.

Lifestyle Changes

Make lifestyle changes;

- Regular exercise. Increase your exercise programme (e.g. build up to 30-60 minutes of power/brisk walking daily, aerobics, swimming and weight-lifting). This will increase HDL and reduce total cholesterol levels. Regular exercise is one of the most important ways of controlling high cholesterol.
- Stop smoking.
- Cut out all forms of coffee, especially unfiltered coffee.
- Drink sufficient water every day (this is based on your weight).
- Reduce alcohol intake to a minimum (e.g. one glass of wine some days).

Dietary Changes

Even though only 10-30% of cholesterol comes from the diet, making dietary changes and making lifestyle changes can be all that is necessary to manage the problem. More than 30% of motivated participants who regularly eat cholesterol-lowering foods under real-world conditions have been shown to lower LDL-cholesterol by 20%, which is not significantly different from the response to a first-generation statin drug[36]. Typical foods eaten in the above trial include **oat bran, oat meal, rolled oats, oat bran breads, barley, psyllium containing cereals, okra, eggplant, soy milk, tofu, soy cheese slices, beans (black, white, kidney), lentils (red, green, yellow), peas (split, black-eyed), Flora Proactiv/Benecol Olive spread, almonds, olive oil, canola oil, skim milk, low-fat yogurt, low-fat cheese, low-fat cottage cheese, white poultry meat (no skin), any fish; lean or extra lean red meats.**

Reduce foods high in cholesterol, e.g. meat, liver, liver patè, kidneys, chicken skin, shellfish (shrimps, prawns), egg yolk and dairy products. Because cholesterol is made in the liver, it is only found in animal products, not in fruit or vegetables. Choose lean cuts of meat and remove the skin from chicken.

Earlier we saw that the total amount of cholesterol we can process in any one day is 1000mg and that the majority of this is manufactured by the liver. However, we do need to reduce the dietary intake as well. The total daily intake of cholesterol in the diet should not exceed 300mg. As an example, one egg can contain 300mg of cholesterol. This does not mean that eggs should be avoided at all costs, but having one egg means that you cannot have anything else with cholesterol in that day. To get an idea of how much cholesterol is in food, look at the following examples.

Food	Cholesterol Content (mg/g)
Chicken Liver	5.61
Chicken Giblets	4.42
Egg yolk	4.24
Beef Liver	3.81
Butter	2.18
Pork Liver Sausage	1.80
Shrimp/Prawns	1.73
Heavy Cream	1.40
Veal	1.34
Pork Ribs	1.21
Lamb	1.21
Pork Shoulder	1.14
Beef Chuck	1.05
Lard	0.94
Crab	0.89

Reduce foods containing the 'bad' fats. These are trans-fatty acids (e.g. biscuits, pastries), hydrogenated oils (most margarines) and saturated fats (animal meats, chicken skin, sausages, bacon, pate, hamburgers, cheese, milk, butter, cream, ice-cream, chocolate, fudge, toffees, cakes, biscuits, pastries, creamy sauces, mayonnaise). Saturated fats are solid at room temperature. Choose low fat cheese, cottage cheese, cream cheese, yoghurts and salad dressings. Instead of butter and ordinary margarine, use spreads that contain monounsaturated fats (olive oil) and polyunsaturated fats. Instead of ice-cream, try Swedish Glace. Use skimmed milk in drinks such as tea, coffee, caffè latte. Eating low-fat foods reduces total cholesterol by 9% [38].

Avoid eating refined carbohydrates (sugar, cake, sweets, biscuits, white bread, crisps, ice-cream, sugar-sweetened drinks).

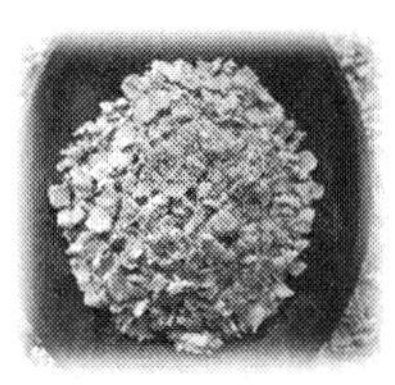

Eat more fibre-rich complex carbohydrate foods (oats porridge, oat bran, barley[37], barley bran, root vegetables, muesli, pulses [e.g. lentils, lentil soup, beans, runner beans, and peas], brown or wild rice, buckwheat, granary bread [wholegrain]). Soluble fibre foods (such as barley) can reduce TC (13-20%)[38], LDL (17- 24%) and TG (6-16%), and increase HDL (9-18%) [37].

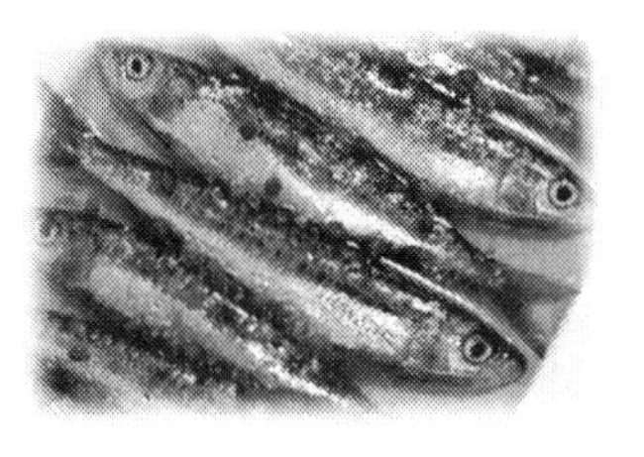

Increase your intake of oily fish. These are a rich source of polyunsaturated fats called omega-3, which ↓LDL. Examples are Wild Salmon (their pink colour is due to Astaxanthin (an antioxidant), which ↑HDL and protects LDL from oxidation), Mackerel, Anchovy, Sardines/Pilchards, Herring, Tuna and Trout.

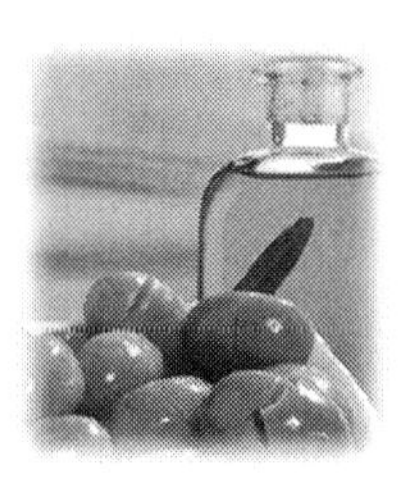

Use plant oils such as fresh linseed oil (without bitter taste), olive oil, canola (rape seed) oil, sunflower oil and safflower oil. These are rich in monounsaturated oils, which can be used for cooking at relatively low heat. Olive oil can be added to salads and food to taste. Canola oil and linseed (flaxseed) oil also contain omega-3. Crushed linseeds can be added to breakfast cereal or porridge.

Eat more fruit, vegetables and nuts (especially walnuts, almonds, pecans and macadamia). Include pomegranate juice, strawberries and avocado pear.

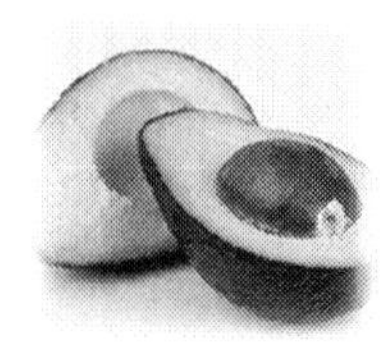

Eat more foods rich in Phytosterols/Phytostanols, structurally similar to cholesterol. They displace cholesterol from intestinal micelles (these deliver cholesterol from the intestines to the bloodstream), thereby reducing absorption. The displaced cholesterol is excreted in the stools. Plants that are naturally high in phytosterols include lettuce, sesame seeds, sunflower seeds, cucumbers, asparagus, okra, cauliflower, spinach, pumpkin, squash, tomatoes, olive oil, celery, and apricots.

Artichoke leaf contains luteolin, which may reduce the manufacture of cholesterol by the liver. One study reported ↓TC (18.5%), ↓LDL (23%), ↓LDL:HDL ratio (20%). In other words, artichokes can improve the ratio of good to bad cholesterol.

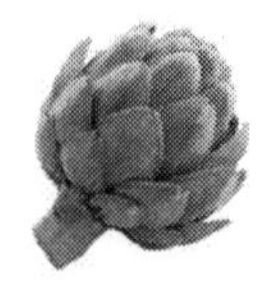

Eat more **garlic** (one clove a day), **onions and tomatoes**.

Shiitake mushrooms contain large amounts of lentinan, a compound which is known to reduce cholesterol levels.

Whole linseeds (flaxseeds) are high on the list of natural high cholesterol treatments because they contain cholesterol lowering omega 3, phytosterols, and are rich in soluble fibre[30]. Linseeds must be ground up or soaked in water before eating because they won't break down during digestion if left whole.

Foods that contain **high amounts of pectin** are good natural high cholesterol treatments. The pectins are mainly found in the fibre of carrots, apples and the white inner layer of citrus rinds. Eating as few as 2 carrots per day may lower cholesterol levels by 10 to 20 percent[30].

Isoflavones. The legumes lupine, fava bean, soy protein, kudzu, and psoralea are excellent food sources for both genistein and daidzein, the isoflavones that can reduce cholesterol[31]. Fermented soya products (tempeh, natto, miso, tofu, pickled tofu [tofu cheese]) - ↓TC (3-9%), ↓LDL (5-13%), ↓Triglycerides (7-10%), ↑HDL (3%), and help to prevent blood clots[32].

Psyllium is type of water-soluble fibre. It also helps prevent constipation. Take 1 tablespoon of crushed psyllium seed and mix in a glass of water, or sprinkle over foods. Psyllium significantly increases HDL[48].

The herb **fenugreek** contains high amounts of a fibre called mucilage, which may lower cholesterol[30].

Curcumin (Turmeric root) can be added to taste, but avoid if you are low in the liver enzyme CYP1A2 (caffeine sensitive people), if you take Warfarin or Propranolol. Also avoid caffeine when taking turmeric. Turmeric attaches to cholesterol and prevents its absorption and it also helps the liver eliminate cholesterol. ↑HDL, ↓LDL and helps keep the blood thin.

Cinnamon (1 to 6g/day) has been shown to ↓TC, ↓LDL, and ↓Triglycerides.

Fennel may reduce cholesterol.

If you wish, drink **one glass of red wine a day**, but be aware that alcohol can cause a rise in both cholesterol and triglycerides.

Both green tea and black tea extracts decrease cholesterol synthesis. Other cholesterol lowering teas are Lime Flower tea, Pu'erh Tuo-Cha tea, Buckwheat tea (buckwheat protein binds cholesterol tightly) and Safflower tea.

Dandelion root tea. Because dandelion is a bitter, it helps to reduce the level of cholesterol produced by the liver[30]. Drink 1 or 2 cups before each meal (or take a tincture three times per day).

Special Cholesterol-lowering Foods (available from supermarkets);

Phytosterols and Phytostanols are structurally similar to cholesterol. They reduce cholesterol absorption, thereby promoting cholesterol excretion in the stools. Two grams a day ↓LDL by 10-15%, ↓platelet aggregation and act as an antioxidant.

Commercial products containing phytosterols/stanols include;

- Lo-Col (vegetable) cheese.
- Flora Proactiv as a spread.
- Benecol products include spread, low fat yoghurt, olive-oil and cream cheese spreads, snack bars and semi-skimmed milk. My favourite is Benecol Olive Spread which contains plant stanols.

Supplements

Always check package inserts of prescribed medication for possible interactions with supplements. This is because natural products can interact with the medication, either enhancing or diminishing its effectiveness.

Major Supplements

Niacin (Vitamin-B3); ↓TC (18%), ↑HDL (20-33%), ↓LDL (10-23%), ↓Triglycerides (26%), ↓CRP and fibrinogen. Possible side-effects: flushing, nausea, liver damage. Niacin appears to be safe and effective in diabetics, despite reports that it may impair glucose tolerance. Don't take with liver disease or raised liver enzymes. Don't take together with statin drugs (the combination may cause rhabdomyolysis). Contra-indicated with Glimepiride and Rosuvastatin. Works well with fibrate drugs for raised triglycerides. Examples; Solgar No Flush 500mg (one at night), Lamberts Nicotinamide 250mg (one or two at night), Inositol Hexaniacinate.

Pantothenic Acid (Vitamin-B5); reduces cholesterol synthesis and increases the burning of fatty acids as an energy source. Useful in Diabetics. Use with caution when taken together with tricyclic antidepressants, e.g. amitriptyline. Side-effects are unlikely at doses less than 1000mg/day, but I have known them to cause headaches in a minority of people. Examples; Solgar 550mg (one daily), Lamberts Calcium Pantothenate 500mg (one daily), Higher Nature's Pantothenic Acid 500mg (one daily with a meal), BioCare's Magnesium Plus Pantothenate (one every evening). ↓TC (19%), ↓LDL (21%), ↑HDL (23%), ↓triglycerides (32%).

Krill Oil 2000mg/day has been shown to ↓TC (18%), ↓LDL (32%), ↑HDL (55%), ↓triglycerides (27%).[18] Due to the blood-thinning properties of krill oil, it is advisable not to take it if you are taking anti-coagulants such as Warfarin (Coumadin) or high-dose aspirin . It is best consult a physician before taking krill oil if you have a seafood allergy, or if you're pregnant or breastfeeding. Krill Oil may cause some side-effects similar to fish oil such as bad breath, heartburn, fishy taste, upset stomach, nausea, and loose stools, but I find the one produced by Cytoplan to be largely free of side-effects. Examples; Cytoplan Krill Oil 500mg, Clean Marine 500mg. Take 1000-2000mg a day, preferably in the morning. Krill Oil remains my favourite supplement for reducing cholesterol levels.

Red Yeast Rice (RYR) also lowers blood pressure. It is made by fermenting the yeast Monascus purpureus over cooked, non-glutinous white rice. It is then sterilised, dried, concentrated and ground. The primary active constituent is Monacolin-K (also called mevinolin, and is an analogue of lovastatin), which inhibits HMG-CoA reductase. This is why RYR is called 'nature's statin drug'. Other cholesterol-lowering agents in RYR are ten other monacolin analogues, omega-3 fatty acids, isoflavones and plant sterols. There is a synergistic action of these multiple components. ↓TC (17%), ↓LDL (22%), HDL remains the same, ↓triglycerides (12%). As RYR is nature's statin drug, always use it together with Coenzyme-Q10. Don't take it if you are allergic to rice or soya, or if you are pregnant or breast feeding[46]. It may interact with some medication, e.g. Amiodarone, certain antibiotics or antifungals, calcium channel blockers (Diltiazem and Verapamil), Cyclosporine, Fibrates. Examples; Solaray 600mg (one twice a day with food), Cytoplan Red Yeast Rice has RYR 400mg, CoQ10 10mg, Hawthorn 50mg (one to three a day, depending on need and effect), Nature's Plus Red Yeast Rice (one twice a day with food).

Garlic capsules (approx 1000mg daily); ↓TC (10%), ↑HDL (31%), ↓LDL (15%), ↓Triglycerides (13%). Examples; Nutri Garlic 6000 (650mg per capsule)(one or two daily with food), BioCare Garlic Plus (one daily with food), Lamberts High Strength Garlic (one daily with food), Higher Nature Garlic Super Strength Supergar (one daily with food), Kyolic 1000mg (one daily). Do not ingest in large amounts for at least 2 weeks before and after surgery as this may interfere with normal blood clotting and may increase bleeding time. Keep doses low in persons with bleeding disorders, such as haemophiliac patients. As it can cause gastric irritation, avoid where there are bleeding ulcers or gastritis. For the same reasons avoid during pregnancy and lactation. Do not ingest garlic in large amounts along with drugs that have anticoagulant activity, such as Warfarin, heparin and aspirin. Use with caution with paracetamol, oral diabetes treatments, insulin injections and thyroid medication.

Viridian Sytrinol 150mg - contains PMFs = polymethoxylated flavones from dried citrus peels, e.g. tangeretin and nobiletin. Take one twice a daily. ↓TC (20-30%), ↑HDL (4%), ↓LDL (19-27%), ↓Triglycerides (24-34%).[16] No special precautions are known.

Berberine has been shown to decrease HbA1c (12%) in diabetics with lipid problems. ↓TC (20-30%), ↓LDL (21%), ↓Triglycerides (36%).[51] Constipation is a known side-effect. Thorne Berbercap 200mg. Take one three times a day.

Minor Supplements

Always check package inserts of prescribed medication for possible interactions with supplements.

Astaxanthin is a potent fat soluble antioxidant from the carotenoid family. It gives the characteristic pink colour to flamingos, salmon, trout, krill, shrimps, prawns and lobster; these eat green microalgae[33]. ↑HDL (10-15%), ↓triglycerides (24%), protects LDL from oxidation, and ↑adiponectin (15-20%).[19] Example; Good Health Naturally AstaXanthin 15mg capsules (one three times a day).

Omega-3 Fish Oils, 3000mg daily (not for epileptics, haemophiliacs or if family history of prostate cancer[23]). These especially ↓Triglycerides, but can increase LDL. Omega-3 and Vitamin-E protect cholesterol from harmful oxidation and from becoming incorporated into the walls of blood vessels. Fish Oil may cause some side-effects, e.g. bad breath, heartburn, fishy taste, upset stomach, nausea, and loose stools. The better the quality, the fewe side-effects. Examples; Solgar 1000mg (three daily), Lamberts Pure Fish Oil 1100mg (three daily), Nutri Eskimo Extra (up to five daily). Fish oils may slightly increase the risk of bleeding in those people taking Warfarin, aspirin or heparin. Care should also be taken with anti-epilepsy medication.

Policosanol (from sugar cane wax); ↓TC (24%), ↓LDL (20-25% in six months), ↑HDL (15-25% in two months), ↓Triglycerides (5%), ↓platelet aggregation and acts as an antioxidant. However, this is the researchers own patent and an independent study failed to find even minimal benefits. Example; Nutri Cholarest SC 10mg tablets (one tablet once or twice a day).

Coenzyme-Q10 (Ubiquinol). Can take months to lower cholesterol. As suggested earlier, it is suggested for people taking statin drugs because statins reduce the synthesis of Co-Q10, thereby inducing fatigue and muscle pain. Examples; Lamberts CoQ10 200mg (one daily), Solaray CoQ10 100mg (one daily), BioCare Co-Q10 Plus (50mg) (one daily). Contra-indicated in those people taking Warfarin.

Turmeric root (Curcumin). Take 900-2000mg of root extract daily. Examples; Lamberts Turmeric 500mg extract, one twice a day. Nutri Inflavonoid 450mg, two twice a day.

Artichoke. Examples; Dr A Vogel Cynara [Globe Artichoke](20 drops in a little water, twice a day), Lamberts Ibisene (16mg cynarin)(two, twice a day with the meals).

Phytosterols. Nutri Sterol-117. Contains phytosterols to trap cholesterol in the gut.

Hawthorn. Take 2000 mg daily in capsule form, or 1 teaspoon of tincture 3 times per day. Example; Solaray 500mg, Solgar 500mg.

Other supplements that may help

- **Ginger**. In addition to lowering cholesterol levels, ginger also temporarily lowers blood pressure. Take one 500 mg capsule three times per day.

- **Fennel**.

- **Inositol hexaphosphate** (IP6).

- **Conjugated Linoleic Acid** (CLA).

- **Vitamin-C**. Take 500 to 1000mg a day.

- **Calcium citrate** 1000mg daily. Brings about a rise in HDL levels.

- **Lecithin**. Has a minimal effect on cholesterol. Higher Nature's High PC Lecithin Granules (one heaped teaspoon with meals, up to 3x/day).

- **Gugulipid/Guggul gum** (extract of commiferous mukul myrrh tree). Theoretically only of benefit in hypothyroidism and poor rate of conversion from T4 (thyroxine) to T3. Nutri's T-Convert (one twice a day with food).

- Works with Water's product called "**help:cholesterol**"[11,12]. This contains the water-soluble fibre Barley Beta Glucan, which reduces cholesterol absorption, ↓TC (9-15%), ↓LDL (9-

15%), but has minimal effect on HDL[35]. Take one sachet (mixed in juice or soya yoghurt) twice a day for a month, then reduce the dose according to results. Beta-glucans are soluble fibres found in cereal such as barley and oats (therefore, not safe for people with gluten allergy or Coeliac Disease). They essentially form a barrier in the stomach which slows down the absorption of fat and sugars produced by the action of bile and enzymes on our ingested food. The loss of bile (which is largely made up of cholesterol) during the digestive process means that more bile must be produced, which results in cholesterol being taken from the blood, resulting in a reduction in blood cholesterol.

- Nutri's **UltraMeal Plus 360**. A meal replacement drink.

- Nutri's **Blackcurrant Seed Oil**. High doses are needed to lower cholesterol.

When discussing the Fasting Lipogram we saw the importance of knowing the levels of total cholesterol, LDL, HDL and triglycerides as well as the ratio of HDL to total cholesterol. We have also seen how different foods and products affect these individual markers.

Which supplements are best?

This depends on what you are trying to achieve as well as the response within each individual. For example, I have found Krill Oil to lower LDL and raise HDL in the majority of patients, but I once had completely the opposite happen. This highlights the importance of checking levels regularly once treatment has been started. I like to re-test the Lipid Profile after three months, then after a further six months if all is well. Once levels have stabilised, annual checks are adequate.

Reducing TOTAL CHOLESTEROL

- Niacin
- Pantothenic Acid
- Krill Oil
- Red Yeast Rice
- Artichoke
- Berberine

Reducing LDL

- Niacin
- Pantothenic Acid
- Krill Oil (avoid fish oils)
- Red Yeast Rice
- Artichoke
- Berberine
- Cholarest

Increasing HDL

- Exercise
- Niacin
- Pantothenic Acid
- Krill Oil
- Garlic
- Calcium citrate
- Psyllium
- Olive Oil

Reducing Triglycerides

- Pantothenic Acid
- Krill Oil
- Omega-3 fish oils
- Niacin
- Astaxanthin
- Berberine

Where to get product – you can get a 10% discount

1. You may try your local health shop or chemist.

2. The Internet.

3. In the UK, most products are available via post from the wholesaler, **The Natural Dispensary**, Tel; 01453-757792. They will need the name of a practitioner. You may use **'DrBrian10'** as a reference in order to get a **10% discount**. If you prefer to order off the internet, go to

www.naturaldispensary.co.uk. Register. Complete the form. There is a box asking for the practitioner. You may use **'Dr Brian'**. At the checkout, put **'DrBrian10'** in the promo box.

Top Tips for reducing cholesterol:

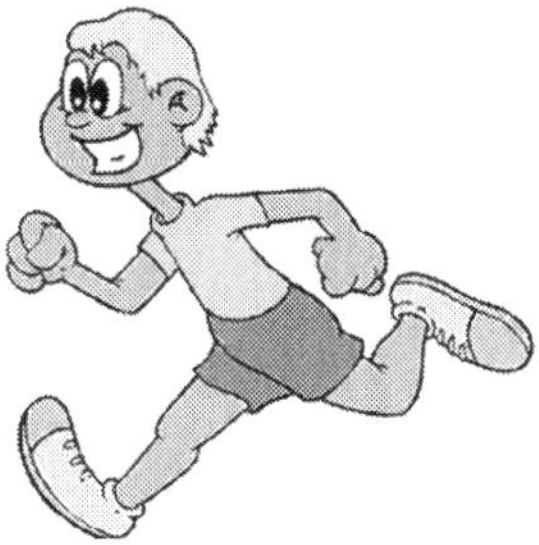

1. Keep your weight at a healthy level.

2. Exercise and keep physically active.

3. Cut down on foods high in cholesterol, saturated and trans-fatty acids.

4. Use more unsaturated fats (plant, seed and nut oils).

5. Eat more wholegrain and fibre-rich foods (pasta, oats porridge, root vegetables, muesli, pulses [e.g. lentils, beans, runner beans, and peas], brown or wild rice, buckwheat).

6. Consider using supplements. Include Co-Q10 if taking a statin drug.

COOKING TIPS

Reduce saturated fat in meat and poultry

Try to consume no more than 170g (six ounces) of cooked lean meat, poultry a day for people who need 2,000 calories. The dietary intake of cholesterol per day should be roughly 300mg. Most meats have about the same amount of cholesterol – roughly 70 mg – in each three ounce cooked serving (about the size of a deck of cards). However, the amount of saturated fat in meats can vary widely, depending on the cut and how it is prepared. Here are some ways to reduce the saturated fat in meat:

1. Select lean cuts of meat with minimal visible fat.

2. Trim all visible fat from meat before cooking.

3. Grill rather than pan fry meats.

4. Use a rack to drain off fat when grilling, roasting or baking. Instead of basting with drippings, keep meat moist with wine, fruit juices or an acceptable oil-based marinade.

5. Cook stews and soups a day ahead of time. Refrigerate when cooled. The hardened fat can then be removed from the top.

6. When a recipe calls for browning meat, use an olive oil spray in a non-stick pan and brown quickly on high heat.

7. Eat chicken and turkey rather than duck or goose, which are higher in fat.

8. Remove the skin from chicken or turkey, preferably before cooking. If you feel that your poultry dries out too much, leave skin on for cooking, but remove before eating.

9. Limit processed meats such as sausages, bologna, salami, hot dogs, lunch meats etc. Many processed meats – even those with "reduced fat" labels – are high in calories and saturated fat. They are often high in sodium as well. Read labels carefully.

10. Organ meats such as liver, sweetbreads, kidney and brain are very high in cholesterol.

Choose Fish at least twice a week

Try to consume no more than 170g (six ounces) of cooked fish or shellfish a day for people who need 2,000 calories. Fish can be fatty or lean, but it is still low in saturated fat. Prepare fish baked, grilled or steamed rather than breaded or fried. Shrimp, prawns, crayfish and crab are higher in cholesterol than most other types of seafood, but they are lower in total fat and saturated fat than most meats and poultry.

Reduce meat in your weekly meal plan

Try meatless meals featuring vegetables or beans. Think of meat as a condiment in casseroles, stews, soups and spaghetti – use it sparingly, just for flavour, rather than as the main ingredient.

Cook fresh vegetables the low-fat, low-salt way

Try cooking vegetables in a tiny bit of vegetable oil, adding a little water during cooking if needed, or use a vegetable oil spray. One to two teaspoons of oil is enough for a package of frozen vegetables that serves four. Tip with mushrooms: they swallow any amount of oil you give them. Once you have put them in with a little oil on a high heat, turn the heat down and cover them to draw moisture and sweat a little.

Add herbs and spices to make vegetables even tastier.

1. Rosemary with peas, cauliflower and squash
2. Mint with peas also works well.
3. Oregano with courgettes.
4. Dill or chives with green beans.
5. Marjoram with Brussels sprouts, carrots and spinach.

6. Basil with tomatoes.

7. Chopped parsley and chives, sprinkled on just before serving. Also enhances the flavour of many vegetables.

Use liquid vegetable oils in place of solid fats

Liquid vegetable oils such as canola, safflower, sunflower, soybean and olive can often be used instead of solid fats such as butter, lard or shortening. Use a little liquid oil to:

1. Pan-fry fish or poultry.

2. Sauté vegetables.

3. Make cream sauces and soups using low-fat or fat-free milk.

4. Make mashed potato with low fat or fat free milk.

5. Use brown rice instead of white rice.

Substitute egg whites for whole eggs

The cholesterol in eggs is all in the yolks – without the yolk, egg whites are a heart-healthy source of protein. Many recipes calling for whole eggs come out just as good when you use egg whites instead of whole eggs. Replace each whole egg with two egg whites. Add a couple of teaspoons of vegetable oil for a moister consistency.

Lower dairy fats

Low fat or fat free milk can be used in many recipes in place of whole milk or use half and half. Some dishes like puddings may result in a softer set. You can also opt for low fat cottage cheeses, Benecol cream cheese (available from Waitrose), low fat mozzarella or goats cheese.

Sauces and gravies

Let your cooking liquid cool, then remove hardened fat before making gravy. Or pop a few ice cubes in the liquid. The fat will stick to them and you can remove it that way. Or, use a fat separator to pour off the good liquid from cooking stock, leaving the fat behind.

Increase fibre and whole grains

1. Use whole-grain bread to make breadcrumbs, stuffing or croutons.

2. Replace breadcrumbs in a recipe with uncooked oatmeal.

3. Serve whole fruit at breakfast in place of juice.

4. Use brown rice instead of white.

5. Use whole-wheat, spelt or buckwheat pasta instead of ordinary pasta.

6. Add lots of colourful veggies to your salad – like grated raw beetroot, shredded raw cabbage and courgettes, etc.

Reduce sodium

Salt is just one source of the sodium we consume every day. Many foods contain sodium in other forms too. Some medicines are also high in sodium. Processed foods and beverages can also be high in sodium. Be aware of all your sources of sodium and aim to eat less than 1,500mg of sodium a day.

1. Use less salt or no salt at the table or in cooking.

2. Use herbs and spices in place of salt.

3. Limit your intake of foods high in added sodium, such as: canned and dried soups, canned vegetables, tomato sauce, mustard, salty snack foods, olives and pickles, luncheon meats and cold meats, bacon and other cured meats, cheeses, take out and some restaurant foods such as French fries, onion rings, hamburgers.

4. To reduce salt in canned vegetables, drain the liquid, then rinse the vegetables in water before eating.

5. Look for "unsalted" varieties of the canned foods and snack foods. Some foods are labelled "no salt", "reduced salt" or "without added salt".

6. Read the labels of foods carefully. Even bakery products and cereals can be a major source of sodium.

7. Ask restaurants not to add salt to your order.

RECIPES

Base mix for a stir fry

Ingredients: (serves 4 people)

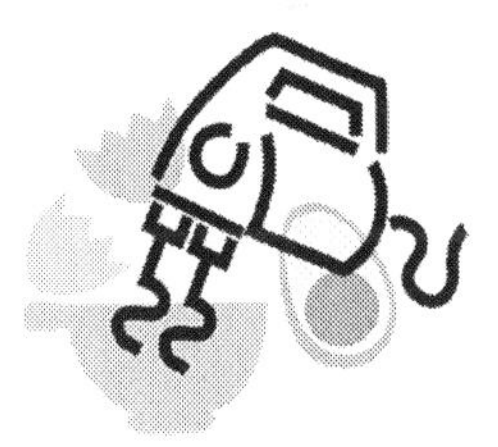

Cook one cup of grains. For example: Half a cup of brown rice and half a cup of barley; or quinoa; or buckwheat or bulgar wheat; or what about a mix of brown rice and green lentils. You can also cook this up adding a stock cube to the pan of water.

2 x small chopped onions (red onion or chopped spring onions work really well or a combination.) Garlic – about two to three cloves mashed up or ready prepared garlic, whatever works best for you.

About 2 -3 cups of chopped vegetables. Make the pieces relatively small as they then cook quickly on the high heat or use baby vegetables. I like to go for a bit of a "crunch" value. Those baby corns are great for that purpose and fresh red or orange peppers. Go for a variety of colour too – so much more interesting. Asparagus is lovely – choose the baby or thin one as then it also cooks quickly. Pak Choi works well too.

1 x tin of beans, chick peas or lentils. I like to use the bean mix in the chilli sauce. (optional)

You can also add any protein you may want to like chicken pieces, Salmon, white fish, thin strips of lean pork or steak, mince etc. If you are adding the chicken or mince raw, then put it into the pan after the onion and garlic. (optional)

Always think "crunch" value – water chestnuts, raw corn cut from the cob, bamboo shoots are all fabulous.

I have also used tofu. What I do is marinade it a bit before in a little pesto or some mild sweet chilli sauce. Then cube it and toss it in to the whole vegetable mix last of all.

Method

Put a good glug of olive oil into your heated stir fry pan. Add the onion and the garlic.

Move the onion and garlic around on a relatively high heat until the onion goes transparent.

At this point add the chicken or meat if it is raw, but not fish if using raw salmon or other fish.

If you are first cooking raw meat or chicken, toss it about in the pan until "sealed" off. In the case of mince let it brown a little. With chicken breast, I really don't like it dry so literally let is just turn pale white and seal off.

Now toss in your vegetables and move around in the base mix until just softening.

If using raw fish it is at this stage that you pop it in. If I am using a piece or two of salmon, I lie it on top and let it steam a little before flaking it up; smoked haddock also works really well. With white fish, flake it a bit first and then toss it in.

Add your tin of beans or pulses (optional). If using the beans in a chilli sauce, then add all of the sauce – it gives it a yummy flavour and work the sauce well into the mix.

Now anything goes for flavour. I use soya sauce, chutney, barbecue sauce, Teriyaki, whatever. Be creative.

The secret is not to lose the crunch value of the vegetables. Enjoy!

Cholesterol-free cake

Ingredients

1 ½ cups all-purpose flour. Any combination of flours will work. You can use ordinary wheat flour, spelt, wholemeal with ordinary flour or it may be a bit dense, rice flour with wheat free flour etc.

¾ cup Xylitol. You can use any form of sugar substitute or brown sugar.

1 ¼ teaspoons baking powder

½ teaspoon bicarbonate of soda

½ teaspoon cinnamon

2 egg whites

1 cup mashed banana
¼ cup of applesauce. If you find that sweetened applesauce makes the cake too sweet, you can leave out the Xylitol or whatever you use to sweeten the cake. Or you can cook fresh apples until they are soft and you have a ¼ cup of apple pulp.

Method

Preheat the oven to 350 degrees.

Lightly grease and flour a cake tin or 8 x 4 inch loaf tin.
In a large bowl sift together the flour, baking powder, **baking soda and cinnamon.

Add the Xylitol.

In another bowl beat the egg whites until fluffy.

Add the bananas and applesauce.

Add the sifted dry ingredients to the wet ingredients.

Pour mixture into the prepared tin.

Bake in the preheated oven for 30-40 minutes until a skewer inserted into the centre of the cake comes out clean.

Turn out onto a wire rack and allow to cool before slicing.

**You can add the baking soda to the wet ingredients and allow it to foam a bit. That can prevent it giving the cake a sharp edge.

Cholesterol-lowering oats porridge

Quantity for One

Heat half a cup of milk (any milk) and half a cup of water

Before it fully boils add a quarter cup of organic jumbo whole rolled oats and a quarter cup of pinhead oatmeal and oat bran mixed. (Half a cup of porridge ingredients altogether)

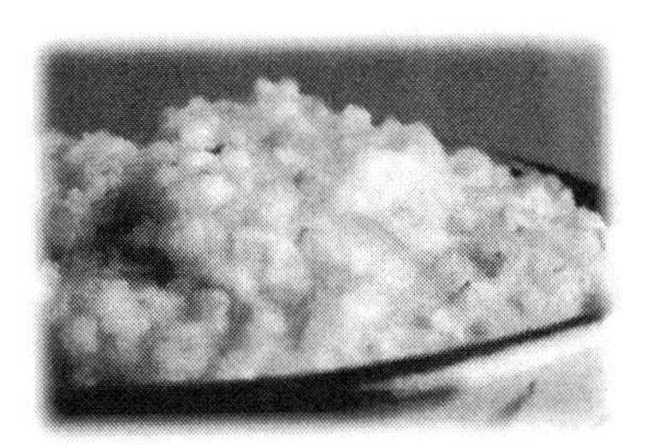

Add a pinch of salt (optional)

When it reaches boiling point, turn the cooker right down and let the porridge simmer for 5-10 minutes. Add a little milk or water is the porridge becomes too stiff.

Eat with cinnamon sprinkled on top. If you like your porridge sweet, then add some agave syrup, Xylitol sugar, honey or brown sugar to taste.

Another yummy option is to cook up some fresh berries – black berries, youngberries, blueberries, cranberries etc. – until they are soft. Sweeten with anything of your choice as mentioned above. Add a tablespoon to your oats with the cinnamon.

Bran Muffin Recipe

Ingredients

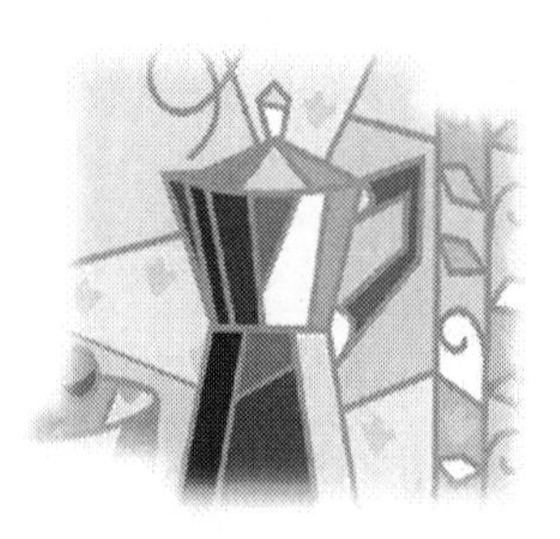

** 2 ½ cups of spelt flour (or other if preferred)

1 cup of Bran (use rice bran or a combination of millet flakes and rice bran if wheat sensitive)

½ cup of oat bran

2 ½ teaspoons of bicarbonate soda

Pinch of salt

2 eggs mixed (use 3 egg whites if you do not want the yolk)

½ cup of vegetable oil –example flora

½ litre of plain yogurt

Instructions

Mix the dry ingredients together and then add the 2 beaten eggs and ½ cup of oil.

Add ½ tub of yogurt

Mix the bicarbonate soda with the rest of the yogurt and wait for it to foam.

Then add to the rest of the muffin mixture.

Leave to stand for 12 hours over night in the fridge.

Preheat the oven for 150-200 degrees Celsius

Oil the muffin tray

Bake in the oven for about 10-15 minutes (or when cooked)

Then enjoy with some sugar fee jam.

**** You can use any combination of flour. Wheat free flours work well too as does a combination of ground**

almond and wheat free flour. You can also combine rice flour, rye flour, polenta, etc.

RESOURCES

1. Pizzorno JE, Murray MT, Joiner-Bey H. The Clinician's Handbook of Natural Medicine. 2nd Ed. Churchill Livingstone, p80-83, 2008.
2. British Heart Foundation. www.bhf.org.uk
3. American Heart Association.
4. American Academy of Family Physicians.
5. Familydoctor.org. Cholesterol: what your level means. Oct 2007.
6. Isaacsohn J. Heart Book. Yale University School of Medicine, 2002.
7. Yang X, et al. Independent associations between low-density lipoprotein cholesterol and cancer among patients with type 2 diabetes mellitus. Canadian Medical Association Journal 2008;179(5):427-437
8. Dr John Briffa, www.thecholesteroltruth.com
9. Ancelin ML, et al. Gender and genotype modulation of the association between lipid levels and depressive symptomatology in community-dwelling elderly (the ESPRIT study). Biol Psychiatry 2010;68(2):125-32.
10. Martinez-Carpio PA, et al. Relation between cholesterol levels and neuropsychiatric disorders. Rev Neurol 2009;48(5):261-4.
11. Center for Metabolic and Endocrine Research, The University of Zulia, Maracaibo, Venezuela. Oat-derived beta-glucan significantly improves HDL Cholesterol and diminishes LDL Cholesterol and

non-HDL cholesterol in overweight individuals with mild hypercholesterolemia. American J Ther. 2007 Mar-Apr;14(2):203-12.

12. Naumann E. Beta Glucan incorporated into a fruit drink effectively lowers serum LDL- cholesterol concentrations. American Journal of Clinical Nutrition, 83(3), 601-605, March 2006.

13. Singh-Manoux, A, et al. Low HDL cholesterol is a risk factor for deficit and decline in memory in midlife: the Whitehall II study (University College London and the INSERM institute in France). Arterioscler Thromb Vasc Biol. 2008 August; 28(8): 1556–1562.

14. Singh-Manoux A. Vascular disease and cognitive function: evidence from the Whitehall II Study. J Am Geriatr Soc. 2003;51:1445–1450.

15. Zureik M, Courbon D, Ducimetiere P. Serum cholesterol concentration and death from suicide in men: Paris prospective study I. BMJ 1996;313:649-51.

16. Sytrinol trials. Quereshi A, Bradlow BA, Brace L, Manganello J, Elson CE, et al. Response of hypercholesterolemic subjects to administration of tocotrienols. Lipid 1995;30:1171-1177. Talbott SM, Roza J, Guthrie N. Effect of citrus flavonoids and tocotrienols on serum cholesterol levels in hypercholesterolemic subjects. Series of studies submitted to Alternative Therapies in Health and Medicine, Boulder CO. www.source-1-global.com.

17. Bratman S. Complementary & Alternative Health. The Science verdict on what really works (in

association with the CMA). Collins 2007, pp 128-131.

18. Bunea R, ElFarrah K, Deutsch L. Evaluation of the Effects of Neptune Krill Oil on the Clinical Course of Hyperlipidemia. Alternative Medicine Review, 2004; 9(4): 420-428.
19. Yoshida H et al. Astaxanthin improves HDL good cholesterol. Atherosclerosis 2010; 209(2): 520-23.
20. Kirby M. Lipid lowering in the ageing population. Geriatric Medicine (GM2), April 2011, 6-9.
21. Doctor Stephen Sinatra. The Coenzyme Q10 Phenomenon. NTC Contemporary Publishing Group, 1998. ISBN 0-87983-957-0.
22. DiMauro S, Quinzii CM, Hirano M. Mutations in coenzyme Q10 biosynthetic genes. Journal of Clinical Investigation, 2007;117(3):587–589.
23. American Journal of Epidemiology. [Men with high DHA from eating oily fish may have an increased chance of developing prostate cancer]. Published online 25 April 2010. http://www.healthfinder.gov/news/newsstory.aspx?docID=652259
24. The Patient Education Institute, Inc. www.X-Plain.com 2008.
25. Harvard School of Public Health, 2009.
26. The Cleveland Clinic Foundation. Stocking a Heart-Healthy Kitchen. 2009.
27. Second Joint Task Force of European and other Societies on Coronary Prevention 1998.

28. Laker MF. Cardiovascular disease prevention: the new Joint British Societies' guidelines. Joint British Societies. 2006.
29. Health Survey for England, 2003.
30. http://www.home-remedy.org/high-cholesterol-treatments.html.
31. Kaufman PB, Duke JA, Brielmann H, et al. A Comparative Survey of Leguminous Plants as Sources of the Isoflavones, Genistein and Daidzein: Implications for Human Nutrition and Health. The Journal of Alternative and Complementary Medicine. Spring 1997, 3(1): 7-12.
32. American Society for Clinical Nutrition. American Journal of Clinical Nutrition, 81(2), 397-408, February 2005.
33. Moyal O. Nature's antioxidant: astaxanthin. Advancing nutrition for Professionals. Higher Nature Issue 4, July 2010.
34. Ose L. Familial Hypercholesterolaemia. An educational booklet for healthcare professionals and patients with familial hypercholesterolaemia. Genzyme cardiovascular, March 2010.
35. Keenan JM, Goulson M, et al. The effects of concentrated barley b-glucan on blood lipids in a population of hypercholesterolaemic men and women. British Journal of Nutrition (2007), 97, 1162–1168.
36. Jenkins DJA, Kendall CWC, et al. Assessment of the longer-term effects of a dietary portfolio of cholesterol-lowering foods in hypercholesterolemia. Am J Clin Nutr 2006;83:582–91.

37. Behall KM, Scholfield DJ, Hallfrisch J. Lipids Significantly Reduced by Diets Containing Barley in Moderately Hypercholesterolemic Men. Journal of the American College of Nutrition, 23(1) 55–62 (2004).
38. Anderson JW, Garrity TF, et al. Prospective, randomized, controlled comparison of the effects of low-fat and low-fat plus high-fiber diets on serum lipid concentrations. Amer J Clin Nutr 1992 56:887-94.
39. Rossebø AB, et al. Intensive Lipid Lowering with Simvastatin and Ezetimibe in Aortic Stenosis. NEJM 2008 Sep 25;359(13):1343-56.
40. Clinical Therapeutics 8(5):537-45, 1986.
41. Minich D. White Paper: UltraMeal with Beta-sitosterol, Sept 2003.
42. Sugrue DD, wt al. British Heart Journal 53, 265-8, 1985.
43. Jansen ACM, et al. Arterioscler Thromb Vasc Biol 25, 1475-81, 2005.
44. Sijbrands EJG, et al. BMJ 322, 1019-23, 2001.
45. Pesonen M, et al. Clin Exp Allergy 2007, Epub ahead of print.
46. Heber D, Yip I, et al. Cholesterol-lowering effects of a propriety red-rice-yeast supplement. American Journal of Clinical Nutrition. 69:2, 231-236, 1999.
47. Dr Uffe Ravnskov. Cholesterol is good for you. CAM, Oct 2011, 30-32.
48. Ziai SA, et al. Journal of Ethnopharmacology. 102 (2), 14 November 2005, Pages 202-207 (Iranian study).

http://www.sciencedirect.com/science/article/pii/S0378874105003983

49. Paul P. Jacques at the Jean Mayer USDA Human Nutrition Center on Aging Tufts University in Boston.
http://www.ars.usda.gov/is/ar/archive/jul95/cholesterol0795.htm?pf=1
http://www.pjstory.com/VitaminCvsStatins.htm
50. Seneff, S. Alzheimer's: a nutritional deficiency disease. CAM, April 2013, 36-38.
51. Yifei Zhang,* Xiaoying Li,* Guang Ning, et al. Treatment of Type 2 Diabetes and Dyslipidemia with the Natural Plant Alkaloid Berberine. J Clin Endocrinol Metab, July 2008, 93(7):2559–2565.

Printed in Great Britain
by Amazon.co.uk, Ltd.,
Marston Gate.